SHIVA BLUE

Strength and Vitality: A Guide to Senior Fitness Over 60

Simple and Effective Workouts to Regain, Maintain and Increase Strength

Contents

Introduction

The process of growing old is inevitable. As we age, our bodies experience discomfort, weakness, and difficulties in maintaining even an upright posture or bending down. Therefore, it becomes increasingly crucial to prioritize our physical well-being and embrace the transformative power of regular exercise.

Welcome to "Strength and Vitality," a companion guide designed to empower seniors over 60 with strength-building exercises tailored to enhance overall well-being. It serves as a guide, a trusted companion on the journey toward optimal well-being emphasizing that the pursuit of fitness is not just a physical endeavor but a holistic approach to living a vibrant and fulfilling life.

The chapters that follow are carefully compiled to address specific facets of senior fitness. From strength and flexibility exercises tailored to the unique needs of aging bodies to nutrition tips that nourish both body and soul, each section contributes to a solid understanding of what it means to thrive in the later years. Practical insights form the core of this book, making it a valuable resource for seniors and those who champion their health.

This book was written by Shiva, your dedicated guide to holistic fitness and well-being. As a seasoned personal trainer and clinical Pilates instructor, she brings a wealth of knowledge and a passion for empowering individuals on their unique fitness journeys. Shiva doesn't just focus on physical prowess; she believes in nurturing a balanced and resilient lifestyle. With a keen eye for individual needs, she tailors fitness plans that not only sculpt bodies but also enhance overall health and vitality. Shiva's approach is characterized by a blend of expertise and empathy, creating a supportive environment where clients feel motivated and encouraged. Whether you're embarking on a fitness journey for the first time or seeking to elevate your current regimen, Shiva is here to guide you with precision, care, and an unwavering commitment to your well-being.

Chapter 1: Understanding Senior Fitness

Welcome to the first chapter of our journey into the realm of senior fitness. In this chapter, we'll investigate the age-related changes that affect muscle strength and vitality, and we'll uncover the importance of strength training for seniors.

Age Related Changes in Muscle Strength and Vitality

1. Loss of Muscle Mass (Sarcopenia) and Its Implications:

- As we age, a natural process called sarcopenia sets in, leading to the gradual loss of muscle mass. This decline, while inevitable, has profound implications for our daily lives. Reduced muscle mass contributes to weakness, making routine activities more challenging and increasing vulnerability to injuries. Understanding sarcopenia is the first step in mitigating its effects through targeted fitness interventions.

2. Decreased Bone Density (Osteoporosis) and Increased Risk of Fractures:

- Another significant change accompanying aging is the decrease in bone density, called osteoporosis or low bone mass called osteopenia. Fragile bones become more susceptible to fractures, posing a considerable risk to seniors, particularly post menopausal women. Understanding the dynamics of bone health is pivotal for implementing strategies that promote bone density, ensuring a resilient skeletal structure that supports an active and independent lifestyle.

3. Impact of Physical Inactivity on Overall Health:

In essence, living a sedentary life is not merely a passive state; it actively contributes to a myriad of health challenges across physical, mental, and metabolic domains. Inactivity disrupts the natural flow of your body.

Let's have a look at what happens when your body, evolved to move is confined to a state of prolonged inactivity.

a) **Cardiovascular Consequences:**

- *Arterial Buildup:* Physical inactivity contributes to the accumulation of plaque in the arteries. This buildup narrows the blood vessels, restricting the smooth flow of blood. Over time, it can lead to conditions like atherosclerosis, increasing the risk of heart disease and stroke.
- *Weakened Heart:* The heart, a powerful muscle, becomes less efficient in a sedentary state. It pumps less blood with each beat, and this reduced efficiency can result in heightened cardiovascular risks.

b) **Metabolic Mayhem:**

- *Insulin Resistance:* A sedentary lifestyle often leads to insulin resistance, where cells no longer respond effectively to insulin. This condition is a precursor to type 2 diabetes, causing an imbalance in blood sugar levels.
- *Weight Gain:* Physical inactivity disrupts the delicate balance between calorie intake and expenditure. With a slowed metabolism, the body becomes prone to weight gain and obesity, further escalating the risk of metabolic disorders.

c) **Musculoskeletal Challenges:**

- *Muscle Atrophy:* The phrase "use it or lose it" rings true in the context of muscles. Inactivity contributes to muscle atrophy, where the size and strength of muscles diminish over time. This not only affects physical appearance but also compromises functional abilities.
- *Joint Stiffness:* Lack of movement can result in joint stiffness. Joints thrive on motion to maintain flexibility and lubrication. Without regular activity, stiffness and discomfort become common issues.

d) **Mental Health Impact:**

- *Cognitive Decline:* The brain, craving stimulation and activity, can experience cognitive decline in a sedentary state. Studies have linked prolonged sitting to an increased risk of neurodegenerative conditions like Alzheimer's disease.
- *Mood Disturbances:* Physical inactivity is associated with mood disturbances and an increased risk of mental health

issues such as anxiety and depression. Exercise is known to release endorphins, the body's natural mood elevators.

e) Digestive Disruptions:

- *Sluggish Digestion:* A sedentary lifestyle may contribute to sluggish digestion. Physical activity promotes healthy digestion by aiding in the movement of food through the digestive tract. Inactivity can lead to issues like constipation and bloating.

f) Weakened Immune System:

- *Compromised Immunity:* Regular exercise is known to boost the immune system. On the contrary, a sedentary lifestyle may compromise immune function, making the body more susceptible to infections and illnesses.

g) Sleep Disturbances:

- *Poor Sleep Quality:* Physical inactivity has been linked to poor sleep quality. Regular exercise promotes better sleep patterns, and without it, the natural sleep-wake cycle may be disrupted, leading to difficulties in falling and staying asleep.

h) Reduced Longevity:

- *Increased Mortality Risk:* Numerous studies have shown that a sedentary lifestyle is associated with an increased risk of premature death. Lack of physical activity is considered a significant factor in various chronic diseases that contribute to reduced life expectancy.

Importance of Strength Training for Seniors

1. Enhancing Muscle Strength and Endurance:

- The cornerstone of senior fitness lies in strength training, a powerful ally against the forces of aging. Engaging in resistance exercises enhances muscle strength, allowing you to tackle daily activities with vigor. As your muscles grow stronger, the ability to endure physical challenges increases, contributing to a more robust and resilient you.

2. Improving Balance and Reducing the Risk of Falls:

- One of the greatest concerns for seniors is the risk of falls, which can have severe consequences. Strength training emerges as a formidable weapon in this battle, as it not only strengthens muscles but also improves balance and coordination. Through targeted exercises, you can build a foundation that safeguards against falls, empowering you to move confidently and securely.

3. Boosting Metabolism and Maintaining a Healthy Weight:

- Metabolism tends to slow down with age, contributing to weight gain and associated health issues such as high blood pressure, type 2 diabetes, body pain and difficulty with physical functioning just to mention a few. Strength training, however, serves as a metabolic booster. By increasing muscle mass, you effectively elevate your resting metabolic rate. This means you burn more calories even at rest, supporting weight management and promoting a healthy body composition.

Closing Thoughts

As we conclude this foundational chapter, it's evident that understanding senior fitness goes beyond acknowledging the changes that accompany aging. It's about proactively embracing strength training as a transformative tool that not only counters the effects of aging but propels you into a life of vitality and independence. In the chapters that follow, we will delve deeper into practical exercises, nutritional considerations, safety measures, and holistic strategies that will empower you on your journey to strength and vitality. Get ready to embark on a transformative adventure that celebrates the resilience and potential within you. Onward to the next chapter of your senior fitness odyssey!

Chapter 2: Preparing for Senior Fitness

Welcome to Chapter 2, where we'll craft your personalized roadmap to strength and vitality. It all begins with understanding your health, consulting with healthcare professionals, pinpointing concerns, and setting achievable goals.

Assessing Individual Fitness Levels

1.Medical Check-Up and Consultation with Healthcare Professionals

- *Why Check-ups Matter:* before diving into any fitness journey, it's crucial to get a health check-up. Think of it as the starting point on your roadmap. Doctors and healthcare professionals can identify potential risks, ensuring you embark on your journey safely.
- *Understanding Your Baseline:* Medical check-ups provide a snapshot of your current health. Blood pressure, cholesterol levels, and other vital markers help create a baseline. This baseline becomes your reference point, allowing you to track progress as you embrace a healthier lifestyle.
- *Consultation for Clarity:* consulting with healthcare professionals isn't just about numbers. It's an opportunity to

discuss your health concerns, ask questions, and gain clarity. Share your goals, any existing conditions, or medications you're on. This collaboration ensures a holistic and safe approach to your well-being.

2.Identifying Specific Health Concerns and Limitations

- *Taking Stock of Your Health:* health isn't just a number on a chart; it's about how you feel and what you can do. Identifying specific health concerns involves an honest self-assessment. Take note of any pain, discomfort, or issues you've been experiencing.
- *Considering Existing Limitations:* we all have our unique set of limitations. It could be an old injury, a chronic condition, or simply a matter of flexibility. Recognizing these limitations isn't a setback; it's a realistic starting point. It helps tailor your fitness plan to accommodate and work around them.
- *Listening to Your Body:* your body often gives signals. Aches, pains, or even moments of fatigue – these are cues worth paying attention to. They guide us in adjusting your fitness routine, ensuring it's a sustainable and enjoyable journey.

3.Setting Realistic Goals for Strength and Vitality Improvement

- *The Power of Realistic Goals:* setting goals is exciting but keeping them realistic is the key to long-term success. Realistic goals are like stepping stones – achievable and motivating. They prevent frustration and keep you on the path to improvement.

- *Breaking Down Your Goals:* instead of aiming for the summit in one leap, break your goals into smaller, manageable steps. If your aim is to enhance muscle strength, start with realistic weight targets and gradually progress. Small victories pave the way for significant accomplishments.
- *Considering Time Frames:* understanding that change takes time is crucial. Rome wasn't built in a day, and your fitness transformation won't happen overnight. Establishing realistic time frames for your goals ensures steady progress without the pressure of unrealistic expectations.
- *Adapting Goals as You Progress:* flexibility is the cornerstone of goal setting. As you progress, your goals might need tweaking. That's perfectly normal. Your body evolves, and so should your objectives. It's a dynamic journey, and your goals should adapt accordingly.

Crafting A Personalized Exercise Plan

1.Incorporating Aerobic Exercises, Strength Training, and Flexibility Exercises

- Aerobic exercises get your heart pumping and your lungs working. Think brisk walking, jogging, or dancing. These exercises are like a heart workout, promoting cardiovascular health. They also help with weight management and boost your overall energy levels.
- Strength training involves activities that make your muscles work against resistance. It could be lifting weights, using resistance bands, or even doing push-ups. This isn't about turning into a bodybuilder; it's about keeping your muscles strong for everyday tasks.

- Flexibility exercises include stretching and movements that increase your range of motion. Think of it as giving your body some extra room to move comfortably. It's not just about touching your toes; it's about preventing stiffness and improving overall mobility.

2.Balancing Intensity and Duration Based on Fitness Levels

- Before diving in, assess your current fitness level. If you're just starting, take it easy. If you're more experienced, you can push a bit harder. The key is to find the sweet spot that challenges you without overwhelming you.
- Intensity is like the spice in your exercise routine. It varies based on how hard your heart is working during aerobic exercises or how much resistance you're using in strength training. Beginners might start with moderate intensity and gradually increase as they get more comfortable.
- How long you exercise is as important as how hard. Start with what feels doable. It could be 20 minutes of brisk walking or a 10-minute strength routine. Over time, aim to gradually increase the duration. Consistency is key.

1. Importance of Warm-ups, Cool-downs, and Proper Form

- Think of a warm-up as your exercise pre-game. It eases your body into the workout, gradually increasing your heart rate and warming up your muscles. It could be a few minutes of light cardio or dynamic stretches. The goal is to prepare your body for the more intense activities ahead.
- Just like a warm-up, a cool-down is the after-party for your muscles. It helps bring your heart rate back to normal and

prevents sudden stops that can make you dizzy. Stretching during the cool-down enhances flexibility and reduces muscle soreness. It's like giving your body a gentle landing after the workout.

- Whether you're doing squats or stretching, doing it right is crucial. Proper form ensures you get the most out of the exercise and minimizes the risk of injuries. If you're unsure, don't hesitate to ask for guidance. It's better to start slow with good form than to rush into it and risk discomfort.

Additional points to consider

If you're new to exercise, begin with simple activities. A 10-minute walk, basic strength exercises, and gentle stretches can be a great starting point. Gradually increase the intensity and duration as you feel more comfortable.

Variety keeps things interesting. Don't stick to the same routine every day. Alternate between aerobic exercises, strength training, and flexibility exercises. It not only challenges different muscle groups but also prevents boredom.

Your body is your best guide. If something doesn't feel right, adjust. Pain is not gain; it's a sign to reassess. As you progress, you'll become more attuned to what your body needs and what feels right.

Closing Thoughts

In this chapter, we've laid out the basics for creating a personalized exercise plan. It's about incorporating aerobic exercises, strength training, and flexibility exercises. Balance the intensity and duration based on your fitness level, and don't forget the importance of warm-ups, cool-downs, and proper form.

Remember, this isn't a one-size-fits-all approach. Your exercise plan should be a reflection of your goals, preferences, and current fitness level. It's a journey, not a race, so let's take it one step at a time toward a healthier, more active you. Onward to the next chapter of your fitness adventure!

Chapter 3: Simple and Effective Strength Exercises

Welcome to Chapter 3, where we dive into the heart of strength training. No need for fancy equipment or complicated routines— just simple and effective exercises tailored for your well-being. You can use dumbbells or standard barbells to execute the exercises.

Let's get started on enhancing your strength, flexibility, and overall vitality.

Tips

- Focus on maintaining proper form throughout the exercise to target the intended muscle groups effectively and to avoid injury.
- Control the speed of both the pulling and releasing phases to enhance muscle engagement and reduce the risk of injury.
- Ensure when using resistance band, it is securely anchored to avoid any accidents during the exercise.

Upper Body Exercises

Engaging in upper body exercises provides a multitude of physical and physiological benefits, contributing to overall health, functional strength, and aesthetic appeal.

1. Biceps Curls and Triceps Extensions:

- *Biceps Curls:* Grab a couple of lightweight objects (could be water bottles, small bags or dumbbells). With arms at your sides, slowly lift the weights toward your shoulders, then lower. This tones those biceps.
- *Triceps Extensions:* Hold a weight with both hands overhead. Bend at the elbows, lowering the weight behind your head while keeping your elbows close to your head, then straighten arms bringing the weight back up overhead. This targets the triceps, the back of your arms.

2. Chest Presses and Shoulder Presses:

- *Chest Presses:* Lie on your back, holding weights above chest. Push the weights upward, then slowly lower them to chest level. It's like giving your chest a friendly workout.
- *Shoulder Presses:* Sit or stand with weights at shoulder height. Push them overhead and bring them back down. This exercise strengthens your shoulder muscles.

3. Modified Push-ups and Chair Dips:

- *Modified Push-ups:* Use a countertop or wall for support. Stand a bit away, lean forward, and push away. This builds upper body strength without the intensity of floor push-ups.

- *Chair Dips:* Sit on a sturdy chair, place your hands on the edge, and lift your body up and down. A great way to work those triceps.

4. Resistance Band Exercises:

Incorporating Band Rows into your resistance band workout routine can contribute to improved posture, increased upper back strength, and enhanced overall upper-body muscle development. As with any exercise program, it's advisable to consult with a fitness professional or healthcare provider to ensure the suitability of the exercises based on individual fitness levels and any existing health conditions.

Begin by choosing a resistance band with an appropriate level of tension.

- *Band Rows:* Secure a resistance band around a sturdy post. Stand facing the anchor point, maintaining a stable and balanced stance with your feet hip-width apart. Hold one end of the resistance band in each hand, keeping your arms fully extended in front of you. Pull the band towards you, squeezing your shoulder blades together. Make sure to keep the band under tension throughout the duration of the exercise.
- *Band Pull-Aparts:* Hold the band in front, arms straight. Pull the band apart, engaging your upper back. Bands provide gentle yet effective resistance.

Lower Body Exercises

Incorporating lower body exercises into your fitness routine provides a range of physical, functional, and health benefits. The lower body is crucial for daily movements, stability, and overall well-being.

Lunges and squats are a versatile and effective lower body exercise that target multiple muscle groups, including the quadriceps, hamstrings, glutes, and calves. These compound movements not only help build strength and muscle tone but also improve balance and stability.

1. Chair Squats and Lunges:

- *Chair Squats:* Stand in front of a chair, slowly lower your body toward it, then stand back up. This exercise targets your thighs and helps with balance.
- *Lunges:* Begin by standing with your feet hip-width apart. Maintain a straight posture, engaging your core muscles. Your shoulders should be relaxed, and your chest should be lifted.

Step forward with one leg, lower your body, then push back up. Lunges work on your thighs, hips, and buttocks. As you step forward, lower your body by bending both knees. The goal is to create two 90-degree angles with your front and back legs. Your front knee should align with your ankle, and your back knee should hover just above the floor without touching it.

Keep your torso upright and your back straight throughout the lunge. Avoid leaning too far forward or backward, as this helps engage the targeted muscles and ensures proper form.

Push through the heel of your front foot to return to the starting position. Use the muscles in your lower body to lift yourself back up. Ensure a smooth and controlled motion throughout the movement.

Repeat the lunge movement on the opposite leg, alternating between legs for each repetition.

2. Leg Raises and Ankle Circles for Improved Mobility:

- *Leg Raises:* While seated, straighten one or both legs and hold in place. Lift the leg(s) a few inches and lower. This strengthens your core and legs.
- *Ankle Circles:* Lift one foot and rotate your ankle clockwise, then counterclockwise. This exercise enhances ankle flexibility and helps with circulation.

3. Step-ups and Seated Leg Extensions:

- *Step-ups:* Use a sturdy step or platform. Step up and down with one foot at a time. This exercise works on your thighs and improves balance.
- *Seated Leg Extensions:* While seated, straighten one or both legs and hold. Lift your leg(s) a few inches and lower. It's a seated version of leg raises.

Core Strength and Stability

Core exercises are crucial for developing and maintaining strength in the muscles of the torso, including the abdominals, obliques, lower back, and pelvis. A strong core is essential for overall health, stability, and functional movement. Here are a few exercises you can incorporate into your fitness routine:

1.   Gentle Core Exercises: Seated Twists, Pelvic Tilts, and Modified Planks:

- *Seated Twists:* Sit with your back straight, twist your torso gently from side to side. This exercise engages your oblique muscles.
- *Pelvic Tilts:* While seated, rock your pelvis forward and backward. It's a subtle movement that strengthens your core.
- *Modified Planks:* Start on your hands and knees, then lift your knees off the ground. Keep your body straight and engage your core muscles by pulling your belly button towards your spine. This will protect your lower back from getting injured. This is a simplified plank that works your core.

2. Emphasizing the Importance of a Strong Core for Balance and Posture:

- A strong core is like your body's anchor. It improves balance, supports your spine, and enhances posture. These simple exercises contribute to a stable and resilient core, vital for daily activities.

Flexibility and Range of Motion

Flexibility and range of motion are essential components of overall physical health and functional movement. These two aspects are closely interconnected and contribute to various aspects of fitness and well-being. Increased flexibility usually increases range of motion.

1. Stretching Routines for Improved Flexibility and Joint Health:

- *Neck Stretch:* Gently tilt your head to one side, bringing your ear toward your shoulder. Hold, then switch sides. This eases tension in your neck.
- *Shoulder Stretch:* Bring one arm across your body, holding it with the opposite hand. Feel the stretch in your shoulder and upper back.

2. Incorporating Yoga-Inspired Movements Tailored for Seniors:

- *Chair Yoga:* Seated or using a chair for support, practice gentle yoga poses. Poses like the seated forward bend or gentle spine twists promote flexibility without strain.
- *Cat-Cow Stretch:* On hands and knees, arch your back up like a cat, then dip it down like a cow. This dynamic stretch warms up your spine.

3.Start Slow, Progress Steady:

- Begin with a few exercises that feel comfortable. Gradually add more as you become accustomed. The goal is progress, not perfection.

- Consistency beats intensity. Aim for regular, manageable sessions rather than sporadic intense workouts. It's about building a routine that sticks.
- If an exercise feels uncomfortable, reassess. It's okay to modify or skip certain movements. Always prioritize comfort and well-being.
- Every step in your fitness journey is a victory. Celebrate your progress, no matter how small. It's these victories that build a healthier, more active you.

Closing Thoughts

In this chapter, we've explored simple and effective strength exercises that cover upper and lower body, core strength, flexibility, and range of motion. The emphasis is on exercises that are accessible, gentle, and beneficial for seniors.

Remember, the journey to strength and vitality is a personal one. Create a routine that suits your preferences and needs. It's not about perfection; it's about progress. So, let's continue this journey toward a healthier, more vibrant you. Onward to the next chapter of your transformative adventure!

Chapter 4: Maintaining and Increasing Strength

Welcome to Chapter 4, where we delve into the secrets of maintaining and increasing your strength. No need for complex strategies; we're keeping it simple and effective. Let's explore the principles of progressive overload and periodization, along with the incorporation of functional exercises for a robust and resilient you.

Progressive Overload and Periodization Principles

1. Gradually Increasing Resistance and Intensity:

- The concept of progressive overload is your secret weapon. It's about gently nudging your body out of its comfort zone by gradually increasing the resistance or intensity of your exercises. If you've been using a particular weight, consider adding a bit more. If you've been walking, pick up the pace or explore inclines. This gradual progression ensures that your muscles stay challenged, fostering growth and improvement.

2. Varying Exercise Routines and Incorporating New Challenges:

- Repetition is good, but variety is the spice of strength training. Switching up your exercise routine not only keeps things interesting but also targets different muscle groups. If you've been focusing on bicep curls, try incorporating lateral raises for your shoulders. If you've mastered chair squats, experiment with step-ups. The idea is to introduce new challenges that stimulate your body in diverse ways.

3. Avoiding Plateaus and Promoting Continuous Improvement:

- Plateaus are like roadblocks on your fitness journey. They happen when your body gets too accustomed to a routine, and progress slows down. By embracing progressive over-load and varying your routines, you can sidestep plateaus. Continuous improvement becomes your mantra, ensuring that every session contributes to the growth of your strength and vitality.

Incorporating Functional Exercises

1. Exercises That Mimic Daily Activities:

- Functional exercises are the superheroes of strength train-ing. They mirror the movements you use in your daily life. Think of them as practical workouts that prepare you for real-world activities. For instance:
- *Squatting:* This mirrors the motion of getting up from a chair or picking something up from the floor.
- *Lunges:* Mimicking the movements involved in walking or

climbing stairs.
- *Pushing and Pulling:* Similar to opening doors or moving objects.

2. Enhancing Overall Strength, Balance, and Coordination:

- Functional exercises aren't just about isolated muscle work; they target multiple muscle groups. This holistic approach improves your overall strength, balance, and coordination. As you lift a bag of groceries or bend down to tie your shoes, your body is better equipped to handle these everyday tasks with ease.

1. Improving Independence and Quality of Life:

- The ultimate goal is to enhance your independence and quality of life. Functional exercises contribute to this by ensuring that your body is well-equipped for the activities that matter most to you. Whether it's playing with grandchildren, gardening, or simply moving around your home comfortably, these exercises pave the way for a more fulfilling and active lifestyle.

Crafting Your Progressive Overload Plan

1. Start with a Baseline:

- Understand where you currently stand. What weights are you comfortable with? How long can you walk without feeling fatigued? This baseline helps in setting achievable goals.

2. Gradual Intensity Increase:

- Once you have your baseline, aim for a slight increase. If you've been doing chair squats, try adding a small weight. If you've been walking, increase the duration or try brisk intervals. Small increments make a big difference over time.

3. Variety is Key:

- Keep your routines dynamic. If you've been focusing on upper body exercises, shift to lower body exercises for a week. Introduce new movements regularly. This not only challenges different muscle groups but also keeps your routine exciting.

4. Listen to Your Body:

- As you increase intensity, pay attention to how your body responds. Soreness is normal, but pain is not. If something feels uncomfortable, adjust or modify the exercise. It's about progress, not pushing yourself to the point of discomfort.

Closing Thoughts

In this chapter, we've uncovered the keys to maintaining and increasing strength for a vibrant and resilient you. By embracing the principles of progressive overload and periodization, we've learned the art of gently pushing our boundaries, introducing new challenges, and ensuring continuous improvement.

The incorporation of functional exercises is a game-changer, offering a practical approach to strength training by mirroring daily activities. As we focus on exercises that mimic everyday movements, we're not just building muscle; we're enhancing overall strength, balance, and coordination. This chapter isn't just about fitness; it's a guide to improving independence and the quality of life. Onward to the next chapter, where we explore holistic approaches to holistic health and well-being.

Chapter 5: Additional Considerations for Senior Fitness

In Chapter 5, we dive into additional considerations crucial for senior fitness—nutrition, hydration, safety precautions, and injury prevention. Let's embark on a journey to understand the importance of a balanced diet, the role of hydration in muscle health, and the significance of safety measures to ensure a thriving and injury-free fitness experience.

Nutrition and Hydration for Optimal Strength and Vitality

1. Importance of Balanced Diet:

- Your body is a reflection of what you feed it with. A balanced diet that consists of protein, carbohydrates, lipids, water, vitamins, and minerals, forms the foundation of optimal strength and vitality. Protein, the building block of muscles, becomes even more vital as we age. Incorporate lean meats, dairy, and plant-based sources like beans and nuts into your meals. Vitamins and minerals, found in colorful fruits and vegetables, play a crucial role in overall health, supporting everything from bone density to immune function.

2. Hydration Guidelines and the Role of Water in Muscle Health:

- Water is the unsung hero of muscle health. Staying adequately hydrated is essential for muscle function, joint lubrication, and overall well-being. Guidelines suggest around 8 cups (64 ounces or 2 liters) of water daily, but individual needs vary. Listen to your body; if you're thirsty, drink up. Water supports digestion, regulates body temperature, and helps transport nutrients to your muscles. It's the elixir that keeps your fitness journey flowing smoothly.

3. Dietary Supplements and Their Potential Benefits for Seniors:

- While a balanced diet is the cornerstone, dietary supplements can offer additional support. Seniors may face challenges in absorbing certain nutrients, making supplements a valuable addition. Calcium and vitamin D, crucial for bone health, are commonly recommended. Omega-3 fatty acids can support heart health, and B-vitamins contribute to energy metabolism. Consult with your healthcare provider to determine if supplements align with your specific needs.

Safety Precautions and Injury Prevention

1. Proper Warm-Up and Cool-Down Routines:

- Before you dive into exercises, your body deserves a warm-up embrace. A proper warm-up increases blood flow to your muscles, enhances flexibility, and prepares your body for the upcoming activity. Gentle cardio, joint rotations, and dynamic stretches are effective warm-up elements. On the flip side, a cool-down is your body's way of gracefully concluding the workout. It gradually lowers your heart rate and helps prevent post-exercise soreness. Stretching during the cool-down aids in flexibility and relaxation.

2. Using Appropriate Equipment and Maintaining Proper Posture:

- The right equipment is like a reliable companion on your fitness journey. Ensure your shoes provide proper support and comfort, especially if you engage in weight-bearing activities. If you're using weights, choose ones that challenge you without straining. Additionally, maintaining proper posture during exercises is a silent protector against injuries. Whether you're lifting weights or doing simple stretches, proper alignment safeguards your joints and muscles.

3. Recognizing Warning Signs and Seeking Medical Attention When Necessary:

- Your body communicates with you, and it's crucial to be fluent in its language. Recognize warning signs such as persistent pain, dizziness, or unusual fatigue. These signals are your body's way of asking for attention. If something doesn't feel right, don't hesitate to seek medical advice. Consulting with your healthcare provider ensures that your fitness routine aligns with your individual health needs and that any potential issues are addressed promptly.

Closing Thoughts

As we conclude Chapter 5, we've navigated the vital terrain of additional considerations for senior fitness. Understanding the importance of a balanced diet, packed with proteins, vitamins, and minerals, is akin to laying a solid foundation for strength and vitality. We've uncovered the significance of hydration, where water emerges as the unsung hero in supporting muscle health. Delving into the potential benefits of dietary supplements has shed light on how these additions can complement a balanced diet for overall well-being. The safety precautions and injury prevention strategies explored, from warm-up rituals to maintaining proper posture, form the bedrock of a sustainable and injury-resistant fitness journey. Remember, fitness isn't just about the exercises; it's a holistic approach encompassing nutrition, hydration, safety measures, and attentive responses to your body's signals.

Conclusion

In concluding this companion guide, we've embarked on a transformative journey toward regaining, maintaining, and increasing strength in the golden years. Throughout the chapters, we've explored simple and effective exercises, importance of assessing fitness levels, mindful nutrition, hydration essentials, and safety measures tailored specifically for seniors. The overarching theme of this guide is not just about physical exercise but embracing a holistic approach to well-being.

Fitness is a personal journey. Your goals may differ from the person next to you, and that's perfectly fine. The focus is on progress, not perfection. Embrace the uniqueness of your journey, relish the improvements, and cherish the newfound strength and vitality.

So, as you conclude this guide, remember that strength training is not just a workout; it's an investment in your overall well-being. The journey to senior fitness is not about reaching an arbitrary destination; it's about creating a lifestyle that fosters vitality and resilience.

Remember, it's never too late to invest in your well-being. Start your journey to strength and vitality today!

If you like my book, please leave a review on Amazon!

Thank you!